CANNABIS AND PREGNANCY:

Navigating the Controversy

Arnold P.

Table of content:

Introduction

- <u>Setting the Stage: Understanding the prevalence of cannabis use and the emerging concerns during pregnancy</u>

Global Trends and Statistics:
Cannabis consumption has experienced a significant surge in recent years, with a notable increase in its acceptance and use across various regions globally. According to the World Health Organization (WHO), about 147 million people, or 2.5% of the world population, consume cannabis annually.
Shifting Societal Attitudes:
There's been a perceptible shift in societal attitudes toward cannabis, particularly with its legalization for medicinal and recreational purposes in several countries and states. This shift has gradually reduced the stigma associated with cannabis use.
Rise in Consumption Among Pregnant Individuals:
Alarmingly, recent studies and surveys indicate a rise in cannabis consumption among pregnant individuals. While specific statistics vary across regions, research shows an increased trend in using cannabis during pregnancy, despite potential health risks.

- <u>Importance of the Discussion:</u>

Maternal and Fetal Health:
- Potential Risks: Understanding and discussing the potential risks associated with cannabis use during pregnancy are essential for safeguarding maternal health and ensuring optimal fetal development.
- Impact on Fetal Development: Addressing the effects of cannabis exposure on the developing fetus is critical in preventing adverse outcomes and ensuring healthy births.

Informed Decision-making:
- Empowering Pregnant Individuals: Open discussions empower pregnant individuals to make informed decisions regarding their health and the well-being of their unborn child.
- Access to Information: Providing comprehensive information enables pregnant individuals to weigh the risks and benefits, making choices aligned with their specific circumstances.

Healthcare Guidance:
- Role of Healthcare Providers: The conversation enables healthcare professionals to offer evidence-based guidance, support, and necessary information to pregnant individuals contemplating or using cannabis.
- Enhancing Patient-Provider Communication: Open dialogue fosters trust and facilitates a supportive environment for pregnant

individuals to seek guidance without fear of judgment.

Ethical Considerations:

- Balancing Autonomy and Health: Discussing cannabis use during pregnancy involves ethical considerations, balancing individual autonomy with the potential risks to maternal and fetal health.
- Ethical Dialogue and Policy Implications: Informed discussions contribute to ethical debates surrounding individual rights, societal responsibilities, and policy-making decisions.

Public Health Awareness:

- Broader Public Health Impact: Understanding the implications of cannabis use during pregnancy on a societal level contributes to public health awareness and policy considerations.
- Minimizing Harm: Addressing this topic helps minimize potential harm by advocating for informed decisions and influencing public health initiatives.

II. The Historical Context and Cultural Perspectives

- <u>History of Cannabis Use: Exploring the historical and cultural aspects of cannabis consumption</u>

Ancient Origins:
- Ancient Use: Cannabis has a rich history dating back thousands of years, with evidence of its cultivation and use across various ancient civilizations like China, India, and Egypt.
- Medicinal and Ritualistic Uses: Historically, cannabis was employed for medicinal purposes, religious rituals, and cultural ceremonies due to its perceived therapeutic and spiritual properties.

Global Spread and Traditional Medicine:
- Spread Across Continents: Over time, cannabis spread to different parts of the world, becoming a staple in traditional medicine and cultural

practices in regions across Asia, the Middle
East, Africa, and the Americas.

- Traditional Remedies: Cannabis was utilized in traditional medicine for treating various ailments, including pain relief, anxiety, and gastrointestinal issues, reflecting its perceived medicinal properties.

Cannabis in Recent History:

- Modern Recognition: The 19th and 20th centuries witnessed increasing scientific exploration and recognition of cannabis's chemical components, leading to its integration into Western medicine.
- Legislation and Social Attitudes: The early 20th century saw a shift in attitudes towards cannabis due to legislative measures, leading to stigmatization and eventual criminalization in many parts of the world.

Counterculture and Medical Cannabis Movement:

- 1960s Counterculture: Cannabis gained popularity as part of the counterculture movement in the 1960s and 1970s, becoming associated with social rebellion and alternative lifestyles.
- Medical Revival: The latter part of the 20th century witnessed a revival of interest in cannabis for medicinal purposes, leading to increased research on its potential therapeutic applications.

Legalization and Current Status:

- Changing Legal Landscape: In recent years, several countries and states have moved towards legalization or decriminalization of

cannabis, both for medicinal and recreational use.
- Cultural Acceptance: Evolving societal attitudes have shifted towards increased acceptance and exploration of cannabis for various purposes, including medicinal, recreational, and wellness-related uses.

- <u>Shift in Perceptions: How societal attitudes towards cannabis have evolved, especially concerning its use during pregnancy</u>

Early Cultural Perceptions:
- Historical Acceptance: Historically, cannabis was viewed in various cultures as a medicinal herb with perceived therapeutic benefits, used for addressing a wide array of health issues.
- Limited Awareness: Early cultural perspectives lacked comprehensive knowledge regarding the potential risks associated with cannabis use during pregnancy.

Changing Perspectives:
- Shift in the 20th Century: The 20th century witnessed a significant shift in attitudes towards cannabis due to evolving scientific discoveries and legislative measures.
- Stigmatization and Criminalization: Cannabis became stigmatized and faced widespread criminalization, affecting public perception and contributing to negative associations.

Contemporary Shifts in Perception:

- Emerging Research Findings: Recent scientific research has shed light on potential risks linked to cannabis use during pregnancy, prompting a reevaluation of societal attitudes.
- Increased Awareness: Greater awareness of potential fetal risks has led to a shift in societal perceptions, emphasizing caution and concerns regarding cannabis use among pregnant individuals.

Healthcare Guidance and Policy Changes:

- Healthcare Recommendations: Healthcare providers have begun cautioning against cannabis use during pregnancy due to emerging evidence of potential adverse effects on fetal development.
- Policy Adjustments: Some regions have updated policies and guidelines to address the risks associated with cannabis use during pregnancy, aiming to protect maternal and fetal health.

Ongoing Debates and Education:

- Continued Discussions: Societal conversations continue, fostering ongoing debates regarding balancing individual autonomy with potential risks to fetal health.
- Education and Awareness Campaigns: Efforts are ongoing to educate pregnant individuals and the broader public about the risks of cannabis use during gestation, emphasizing informed decision-making.

The evolution of societal attitudes towards cannabis and pregnancy reflects a shift from historical acceptance to modern-day caution due to increased awareness of potential risks backed by scientific research. This shift highlights the importance of healthcare guidance, policy adjustments, ongoing discussions, and educational initiatives in shaping contemporary perceptions and promoting informed decision-making among pregnant individuals regarding cannabis use.

III. *Cannabis and the Pregnant Body*

- <u>Biological Impact: Understanding how cannabinoids interact with the body during pregnancy</u>

Endocannabinoid System (ECS) Overview:
- Natural System: The ECS is a complex biological system present in humans, involving cannabinoid receptors, endocannabinoids (naturally occurring compounds), and enzymes.
- Regulatory Role: It plays a crucial role in regulating various physiological processes, including mood, appetite, pain sensation, and reproductive functions.

Interaction of Cannabinoids with the ECS:
- Cannabinoid Reception: Cannabinoids from cannabis plants, such as THC (tetrahydrocannabinol) and CBD (cannabidiol), interact with the ECS by binding to cannabinoid receptors (CB1 and CB2) in the body.
- Impact on Signaling: These cannabinoids alter neurotransmitter release, affecting signal

transmission in the brain and body, thereby influencing various bodily functions.

Placental Development and Pregnancy:

- Placental Function: During pregnancy, the placenta plays a vital role in supplying nutrients and oxygen to the developing fetus while removing waste products.
- Cannabinoid Impact: Research suggests that cannabinoids can affect placental development by influencing blood flow, nutrient transport, and hormone production, potentially impacting fetal growth and development.

Risks Associated with Cannabinoid Exposure:

- Fetal Neurodevelopment: Cannabinoid exposure during gestation can potentially disrupt normal fetal brain development due to the influence on neurotransmitter systems.
- Potential Outcomes: Studies indicate potential risks, such as impaired cognitive function, altered behavior, and increased susceptibility to neurodevelopmental disorders in offspring exposed to cannabinoids during pregnancy.

Variability and Dose-Dependent Effects:

- Differential Impact: The impact of cannabinoids on pregnancy outcomes may vary based on factors such as the timing of exposure, dosage, frequency, and individual differences.
- Challenges in Research: Establishing precise dosage thresholds and effects remains challenging due to limited research and the complexity of biological interactions.

Understanding how cannabinoids interact with the body's ECS during pregnancy sheds light on their potential impact on placental development and fetal neurodevelopment. This biological insight forms a crucial foundation for assessing the potential risks associated with cannabinoid exposure during gestation and highlights the need for further research to elucidate the precise effects and dosage thresholds for pregnant individuals.

- <u>Review of Studies: Summarizing existing research and the scientific understanding of cannabis effects on gestation</u>

Existing Research Findings:
- Diverse Studies: Multiple scientific investigations have explored the effects of cannabis use during pregnancy on maternal and fetal health outcomes.
- Variability in Findings: Studies have presented a spectrum of findings, reflecting varying methodologies, populations studied, and differing approaches to measuring cannabis exposure.

Maternal Health Outcomes:
- Adverse Pregnancy Outcomes: Several studies have associated cannabis use during pregnancy with an increased risk of adverse outcomes,

including stillbirths, preterm births, and low birth weights.

- Maternal Complications: Research also suggests potential links between cannabis use and maternal complications, such as gestational hypertension and altered placental development.

Fetal Development and Long-term Impact:

- Neurodevelopmental Concerns: Evidence indicates a potential association between maternal cannabis use and altered neurodevelopment in offspring, potentially impacting cognitive functions and behavior.
- Long-term Consequences: Some studies suggest a higher likelihood of neurobehavioral issues and developmental disorders in children exposed to cannabis in utero.

Dosage and Timing Considerations:

- Dose-Dependent Effects: Research suggests that the impact of cannabis on gestation outcomes may be influenced by dosage, frequency, and timing of exposure during pregnancy.
- Varied Findings: Conflicting findings exist regarding specific dosage thresholds and the extent of effects based on the timing of cannabis use during gestation.

Research Limitations and Gaps:

- Challenges in Studying Cannabis: Ethical and methodological constraints pose challenges in conducting controlled studies due to legal implications and the complexity of isolating cannabis use from other variables.

- Need for Further Investigation: Existing research gaps necessitate more extensive and controlled studies to establish clearer causal relationships and better understand the comprehensive effects of cannabis on gestational outcomes.

The existing body of research presents diverse findings regarding the effects of cannabis use during pregnancy on maternal and fetal health. While several studies suggest associations between cannabis use and adverse outcomes, variability in findings and research limitations underscore the need for more rigorous and controlled investigations to elucidate the precise impacts and establish clearer causal relationships between cannabis use during gestation and its effects on maternal and fetal health.

IV. Unpacking the Risks and Adverse Outcomes

- <u>Adverse Effects: Exploring potential risks associated with cannabis use during pregnancy</u>

Impact on Fetal Development:
- Neurodevelopmental Concerns: Studies suggest a potential association between maternal cannabis use and altered brain development in the fetus, leading to cognitive and behavioral issues in offspring.
- Risk of Impaired Cognition: Prenatal exposure to cannabinoids might affect neurodevelopmental processes, potentially contributing to learning difficulties or attention-related problems in children.

Adverse Pregnancy Outcomes:
- Preterm Birth: Research indicates an increased likelihood of preterm birth among pregnant individuals who use cannabis, leading to potential health complications for the newborn.
- Low Birth Weight: Maternal cannabis use during pregnancy might correlate with a higher incidence of delivering infants with lower than average birth weight, which can pose health risks to the baby.

Placental and Maternal Health:

- Placental Abnormalities: Cannabis use may impact placental function, potentially leading to alterations in nutrient exchange, blood flow, and hormone regulation, affecting fetal growth and development.
- Hypertensive Disorders: Studies suggest a potential association between cannabis use and an increased risk of gestational hypertension, posing health risks to both the mother and the fetus.

Long-term Behavioral and Cognitive Impact:
- Behavioral Issues: Exposure to cannabis during gestation might increase the risk of behavioral problems, such as impulsivity, hyperactivity, and attention deficits in children.
- Cognitive Function: Prenatal cannabis exposure might affect cognitive functions in offspring, potentially influencing learning abilities and intellectual development.

Variability and Dose-Dependent Effects:
- Differential Impact: The severity of potential risks could vary based on factors such as the frequency, dosage, duration, and timing of cannabis use during pregnancy.
- Complexity in Research: Determining precise thresholds or establishing clear causal relationships between dosage and outcomes remains challenging due to limited controlled studies and the complex nature of human responses.

Exploring the potential risks associated with cannabis use during pregnancy reveals concerns related to fetal neurodevelopment, adverse pregnancy outcomes, placental health, and long-term cognitive and behavioral impacts on offspring. While research suggests associations, understanding the precise extent and causality of these risks necessitates further comprehensive studies to better inform healthcare guidance and support for pregnant individuals.

- <u>Impact on Fetal Development: Understanding how cannabis consumption affects the unborn child</u>

Neurodevelopmental Concerns:
- Brain Development: Cannabis compounds, particularly THC, can cross the placenta and reach the fetal brain, potentially interfering with crucial neurodevelopmental processes.
- Potential Disruptions: Exposure to cannabinoids during gestation might impact the formation of neuronal circuits, altering the structure and function of the developing brain.

Cognitive and Behavioral Outcomes:
- Risk of Cognitive Impairment: Studies suggest a link between maternal cannabis use and cognitive deficits in offspring, potentially affecting learning, memory, and information processing abilities.
- Behavioral Issues: Prenatal exposure to cannabinoids could contribute to behavioral

problems in children, such as impulsivity, hyperactivity, and attention-related difficulties.

Vulnerability of Developing Systems:

- Sensitive Developmental Periods: Fetal brains undergo critical periods of growth and differentiation, making them susceptible to external influences, including cannabinoids.
- Potential Long-term Impact: Cannabis exposure during gestation might lead to persistent changes in brain structure or function, impacting the child's behavior and cognitive abilities in later life stages.

Placental and Physiological Changes:

- Placental Effects: Cannabis use may affect the placenta's function, disrupting the exchange of nutrients, oxygen, and waste products between the mother and fetus.
- Hormonal and Physiological Alterations: Cannabinoids might interfere with hormonal signaling pathways, influencing fetal growth and development, potentially leading to adverse outcomes.

Variability in Impact:

- Individual Variations: The impact of cannabis on fetal development might vary among individuals due to genetic predispositions, maternal health factors, and varying levels of cannabinoid exposure.
- Complexity in Research: Determining precise mechanisms and establishing clear causal relationships between cannabis exposure and specific fetal developmental outcomes remains

a challenge due to the multifaceted nature of
human biology.

V. Strategies for Mitigating Risks and Safer Alternatives

- <u>Risk Reduction Techniques: Practical guidance for pregnant individuals to minimize cannabis-related risks</u>

Abstain from Cannabis Use:
- Complete Abstinence: The safest approach is to avoid cannabis use entirely during pregnancy to eliminate potential risks associated with exposure to cannabinoids.

Seek Alternative Therapies:
- Consult Healthcare Providers: Discuss with healthcare professionals to explore alternative therapies or medications that are safe and approved for managing pregnancy-related symptoms.
- Non-Pharmacological Options: Consider non-pharmacological methods such as relaxation techniques, dietary modifications, or prenatal exercises to alleviate discomfort.

Open Communication:
- Honest Conversations: Have open and transparent discussions with healthcare providers about any previous or ongoing cannabis use to receive appropriate guidance and support.
- Non-Judgmental Environment: Seek healthcare providers who offer a supportive and non-judgmental atmosphere to address concerns without fear of reproach.

Establish a Support System:

- Social Support: Build a support network comprising family, friends, or support groups to navigate through pregnancy challenges without resorting to cannabis use.
- Seeking Help: Encourage seeking help or counseling if dealing with stress, anxiety, or other conditions that may trigger the temptation to use cannabis.

Education and Resources:

- Access Reliable Information: Equip oneself with reliable resources and educational materials about the potential risks of cannabis use during pregnancy.
- Stay Informed: Regularly seek updated information from credible sources and stay aware of any new research findings on the subject.

Self-care Practices:

- Healthy Lifestyle: Prioritize a healthy lifestyle encompassing balanced nutrition, regular exercise, and adequate rest to support overall well-being during pregnancy.
- Stress Management: Employ stress-relief techniques like mindfulness, meditation, or prenatal yoga to manage stress without resorting to cannabis.

By prioritizing complete abstinence, seeking alternative therapies under professional guidance, fostering open communication with healthcare providers, building a support network, staying informed, practicing self-care, and managing stress through healthy means, pregnant individuals can actively reduce potential risks associated with cannabis use during gestation, safeguarding maternal and fetal health.

- <u>Safer Alternatives: Exploring alternative methods to manage pregnancy symptoms without cannabis</u>

Nausea and Vomiting:
- Ginger: Ginger tea or supplements can alleviate nausea; try ginger ale or ginger chews for relief.
- Small, Frequent Meals: Eating smaller, more frequent meals can help manage nausea and prevent vomiting.
- Acupressure Bands: Wristbands designed for acupressure, like Sea-Bands, might provide relief from nausea.

Pain Relief and Discomfort:
- Physical Therapy: Seek guidance from a physical therapist for exercises or stretches to ease discomfort, particularly in the back or hips.
- Heat or Cold Packs: Applying heat or cold packs to areas of discomfort can provide relief from muscle aches or joint pains.
- Maternity Support Belts: Supportive belts designed for pregnancy can help alleviate back pain by providing additional support.

Anxiety and Stress Management:

- Mindfulness and Relaxation Techniques: Practice deep breathing exercises, meditation, or prenatal yoga to reduce stress and anxiety.
- Counseling or Therapy: Consider seeking professional counseling or therapy to address emotional concerns and stress management during pregnancy.
- Support Groups: Joining pregnancy support groups or classes can provide a sense of community and emotional support.

Sleep Difficulties:

- Sleep Hygiene: Maintain a regular sleep schedule, create a comfortable sleep environment, and practice relaxation techniques before bedtime.
- Body Pillows: Use pregnancy-specific body pillows to find a more comfortable sleeping position and support body alignment.

Heartburn and Indigestion:

- Dietary Adjustments: Avoiding spicy and fatty foods, eating smaller meals, and avoiding lying down right after eating can help reduce heartburn.
- Elevating Head while Sleeping: Prop yourself up with extra pillows to keep your head elevated while sleeping to alleviate nighttime heartburn.

VI. *Public Health, Policy, and Healthcare Recommendations*

- <u>Public Health Implications: Examining the broader implications for public policy and health initiatives</u>

Policy Frameworks:
- Regulatory Measures: Policy decisions need to consider the balance between individual autonomy and public health concerns.
- Legislation and Guidelines: Developing clear policies and guidelines that address the risks of cannabis use during pregnancy while respecting individual rights is crucial.

Healthcare Practices:
- Healthcare Guidelines: Standardizing healthcare recommendations and protocols to discourage cannabis use during gestation is essential.
- Professional Training: Healthcare providers require comprehensive training to offer informed guidance and support to pregnant individuals regarding cannabis use.

Public Awareness and Education:
- Information Dissemination: Implementing educational campaigns to raise awareness among pregnant individuals and the general public about the risks associated with cannabis during pregnancy.
- Accessible Resources: Providing easily accessible, evidence-based resources to

empower informed decision-making among pregnant individuals.

Research and Data Collection:

- Continued Research: Encouraging further research to bridge existing gaps in understanding the precise impacts of cannabis use during pregnancy.
- Data Collection Efforts: Facilitating comprehensive data collection initiatives to better understand trends and prevalence rates of cannabis use in pregnant populations.

Ethical Considerations:

- Autonomy vs. Public Health: Balancing individual autonomy with the need to protect maternal and fetal health raises ethical dilemmas in policymaking.
- Social Equity: Addressing disparities in access to information and resources, ensuring equitable support for pregnant individuals from diverse backgrounds.

Collaborative Efforts:

- Interdisciplinary Collaboration: Fostering collaboration among policymakers, healthcare professionals, researchers, and advocacy groups to formulate holistic strategies.
- Community Engagement: Involving communities in discussions and decision-making processes to ensure policies reflect diverse perspectives and needs.

Addressing the public health implications of cannabis use during pregnancy necessitates comprehensive policy frameworks, healthcare practices, public education initiatives, continued research efforts, ethical considerations, and collaborative approaches. Establishing a balance between individual rights, public health interests, and equitable support for pregnant individuals is critical in shaping effective policies and health initiatives.

- <u>Healthcare Guidelines: Recommendations for healthcare providers and their role in advising pregnant individuals</u>

Healthcare Provider Guidelines:

Informed and Non-Judgmental Approach:

- Education and Guidance: Offer comprehensive and evidence-based information regarding the potential risks of cannabis use during pregnancy.
- Non-Judgmental Environment: Create a supportive atmosphere that encourages open dialogue without stigmatizing or condemning pregnant individuals for their past or present cannabis use.

Establishing Clear Communication:

- Open Discussions: Initiate conversations early during prenatal care visits, inquiring about any history or current use of cannabis.
- Encouraging Honesty: Assure confidentiality and emphasize the importance of honest disclosure to provide appropriate guidance.

Provision of Evidence-based Information:

- Risks and Benefits: Educate pregnant individuals about the potential risks associated with cannabis use during gestation, emphasizing its impact on fetal development and pregnancy outcomes.
- Alternative Strategies: Offer alternative, safe, and evidence-backed approaches to manage pregnancy-related symptoms without resorting to cannabis.

Individualized Support and Care:
- Tailored Guidance: Recognize individual circumstances and needs while providing personalized guidance and support.
- Referral to Support Services: Offer referrals to counseling, addiction services, or specialized care for individuals facing challenges related to cannabis use during pregnancy.

Continuous Education and Training:
- Continual Update: Stay updated with the latest research findings, guidelines, and policy changes related to cannabis use during pregnancy.
- Training and Professional Development: Participate in training programs or workshops to enhance knowledge and skills in addressing this complex issue effectively.

Collaboration and Multidisciplinary Approach:
- Team-based Care: Collaborate with other healthcare professionals, including obstetricians, counselors, and addiction specialists, to offer comprehensive care.
- Community Resources: Be aware of and refer pregnant individuals to community resources

that provide support for substance use disorders or pregnancy-related concerns.

VII.Beyond the Study: Unanswered Questions and Future Directions

- <u>Research Gaps: Highlighting areas requiring further investigation and understanding</u>

Long-term Effects on Offspring:
- Comprehensive Longitudinal Studies: There's a need for extensive longitudinal studies assessing the long-term neurodevelopmental outcomes in children exposed to cannabis during gestation.
- Cognitive and Behavioral Impact: Further exploration is required to understand the lasting cognitive, behavioral, and socio-emotional effects in children as they progress through different developmental stages.

Placental Function and Mechanisms:
- Placental Biology: Investigating the specific mechanisms through which cannabinoids affect placental function, hormone regulation, and nutrient transport during pregnancy is crucial.
- Differentiation of Effects: Understanding how various components of cannabis, including THC and CBD, affect placental development and function differently.

Dosage and Timing Effects:
- Dose-Response Relationships: Establishing clear dose-response relationships to determine thresholds of exposure and their impact on maternal and fetal health outcomes.
- Timing of Exposure: Investigating how the timing of cannabis exposure during gestation

influences different developmental stages and outcomes.

Biomarkers and Detection Methods:

- Improved Detection Techniques: Developing more accurate and efficient biomarkers or detection methods for assessing cannabis exposure during pregnancy.
- Distinguishing Cannabis Products: Differentiating between various cannabis products (e.g., THC-dominant strains, CBD products) in determining their differential impacts on pregnancy outcomes.

Health Disparities and Sociocultural Factors:

- Inclusivity in Research: Addressing disparities in research representation to encompass diverse populations and their unique sociocultural contexts.
- Impact of Social Factors: Understanding the interplay of societal factors, socioeconomics, and cultural norms on cannabis use behavior and its effects during pregnancy.

Intervention Strategies and Support:

- Efficacy of Interventions: Evaluating the effectiveness of intervention programs designed to support pregnant individuals in cessation or harm reduction regarding cannabis use.
- Identifying Protective Factors: Identifying protective factors or resources that mitigate the risks associated with cannabis use during gestation.

Short-term Effects on offspring:

- Neurodevelopmental Impact: Potential short-term changes in neurobehavioral patterns, such as altered stress response or differences in motor development.
- Impaired Neurocognition: Short-term effects may manifest as subtle cognitive differences, affecting attention or early learning abilities in some children.
- Birth Outcomes: Immediate effects may include a slightly increased risk of low birth weight or potential alterations in early infant behavior.
- Neonatal Adaptation: Infants exposed to cannabis might display subtle differences in neonatal behavior, such as tremors or alterations in visual responsiveness, although these effects tend to be transient.

It's important to note that while short-term effects have been observed in some studies, further research is needed to elucidate the precise extent and duration of these effects on offspring following maternal cannabis use during pregnancy.

- <u>Future Research Directions: Suggestions for future studies and inquiries into the subject</u>

Future Research Directions:
Longitudinal Studies:

- Extended Follow-ups: Conduct comprehensive longitudinal studies tracking children exposed to maternal cannabis use from gestation through adolescence and adulthood to assess long-term outcomes.
- Multigenerational Impact: Investigate potential multigenerational effects by examining the offspring of individuals who were exposed to cannabis during their own gestation.

Mechanistic Investigations:

- Placental Function: Explore in-depth the specific mechanisms through which cannabinoids influence placental development and function, considering different cannabinoid constituents and their effects.
- Neurobiological Underpinnings: Investigate the neurobiological underpinnings of cannabinoid exposure on fetal brain development and explore the impact on specific neural pathways.

Dose and Timing Effects:

- Dose-Response Relationships: Establish clear dose-response relationships to ascertain thresholds of exposure and their effects on various developmental domains.
- Timing-Specific Impacts: Examine the differential impacts of cannabis exposure during different trimesters or critical developmental windows on offspring outcomes.

Biomarkers and Detection:

- Improved Detection Methods: Develop more sensitive and specific biomarkers or detection methods for assessing cannabis exposure during pregnancy accurately.

- Distinguishing Cannabis Types: Investigate the differential effects of various cannabis constituents and strains, distinguishing between THC-dominant and CBD-rich products.

Intervention Strategies:

- Efficacy of Interventions: Assess the effectiveness of interventions and support programs aimed at reducing or preventing cannabis use during pregnancy.
- Tailored Support Approaches: Identify and evaluate personalized or culturally sensitive approaches to support pregnant individuals in managing cannabis use and reducing potential risks.

Health Disparities and Contextual Factors:

- Diversity in Research: Focus on inclusivity in research to understand how diverse sociocultural contexts and disparities influence cannabis use behavior and its effects during pregnancy.
- Socioeconomic Impact: Investigate the interplay between socioeconomic factors, mental health, and access to resources concerning cannabis use and its outcomes during gestation.

Addressing these future research directions will contribute significantly to a deeper understanding of the complexities surrounding maternal cannabis use during pregnancy. Advancements in these areas will aid in refining healthcare guidance, formulating effective interventions, and shaping policies that prioritize the well-being of both pregnant individuals and their offspring.

VIII.Real-life Narratives and Perspectives

- <u>Expert Insights: Perspectives from healthcare professionals, researchers, and specialists</u>

Perspectives from Healthcare Professionals, Researchers, and Specialists:

Healthcare Provider Perspective:

- Emphasis on Abstinence: Healthcare providers generally advocate for complete abstinence from cannabis during pregnancy due to potential risks identified in existing research.
- Balancing Support and Education: They focus on providing non-judgmental support and comprehensive education to pregnant individuals, emphasizing the potential risks to maternal and fetal health.

Researcher Insights:

- Call for Further Studies: Researchers stress the need for more rigorous and controlled studies to elucidate causal relationships and the

specific impacts of cannabis use on gestational outcomes.
- Multifaceted Research Approaches: They advocate for multifaceted research approaches that explore mechanistic insights, dosage effects, and long-term developmental consequences on offspring.

Specialist Standpoint:
- Risk Mitigation Strategies: Specialists likely highlight the importance of developing and evaluating interventions aimed at mitigating risks associated with cannabis use during pregnancy.
- Individualized Care: They might emphasize the need for tailored approaches considering individual circumstances, recognizing that one size doesn't fit all in addressing this issue.

Healthcare professionals, researchers, and specialists often align in their emphasis on caution regarding cannabis use during pregnancy due to potential risks. They advocate for evidence-based guidance, continual research efforts, and personalized approaches to support pregnant individuals and protect maternal and fetal health. Their insights collectively highlight the importance of comprehensive strategies and ongoing research to address this complex issue effectively.

IX. Conclusion: Empowering Informed Choices

- <u>Summarising Insights: Recapitulating key learnings and significant takeaways from the book</u>

Summary of Key Insights:

1. Risks and Impact on Offspring:
   - Maternal cannabis use during pregnancy poses potential risks to fetal development and birth outcomes, influencing neurodevelopment and possibly leading to cognitive and behavioral changes in offspring.
2. Placental Function and Health:
   - Cannabis exposure may impact placental function, contributing to alterations in nutrient exchange and hormone regulation, affecting fetal growth and development.
3. Short and Long-term Effects:
   - Both short-term and potential long-term effects on offspring, such as altered neurocognition, behavioral differences, and potential developmental challenges, warrant continued investigation.
4. Complexity in Research Findings:
   - Existing research exhibits variability in findings, emphasizing the need for clearer dose-response relationships, precise timing effects, and distinguishing impacts based on cannabis constituents.
5. Healthcare Guidance and Support:
   - Healthcare providers play a pivotal role in offering evidence-based guidance, establishing open communication, and providing non-

judgmental support to pregnant individuals
regarding cannabis use.

6. Public Health Implications and Policies:
- Addressing the public health implications involves creating clear policies, standardized healthcare practices, and public education to raise awareness about the risks associated with cannabis use during pregnancy.

7. Future Research Directions:
- Ongoing research needs to focus on longitudinal studies, mechanistic investigations, dose and timing effects, improved detection methods, and considering social and contextual factors to address current gaps in understand.

The comprehensive exploration of maternal cannabis use during pregnancy reveals potential risks, ranging from placental function to neurodevelopmental impacts on offspring. The complexity in research findings underscores the need for clearer guidance, robust policies, continual research efforts, and supportive healthcare practices to safeguard maternal and fetal well-being. Further research is crucial to refine our understanding and guide strategies aimed at minimizing risks associated with cannabis use during gestation.

1.Access to Comprehensive Information:
- Encourage pregnant individuals to seek comprehensive, evidence-based information from reliable sources about the potential risks and effects of cannabis use during gestation.

2. Open Communication with Healthcare Providers:
- Advocate for open and honest discussions with healthcare providers to understand individual risks, receive tailored guidance, and make informed choices regarding cannabis use.

3. Exploration of Alternative Strategies:
- Empower pregnant individuals to explore and discuss alternative, safer methods for managing pregnancy-related symptoms without resorting to cannabis.

4. Understanding Individual Contexts:
- Highlight the importance of recognizing individual circumstances, including personal health history, lifestyle, and specific needs, in making decisions concerning cannabis use during pregnancy.

5. Supportive Environments and Community Resources:
- Encourage seeking support from healthcare professionals, community resources, or support groups that offer non-judgmental guidance and assistance in navigating pregnancy-related challenges.

6. Stress on Personal Autonomy and Well-being:

- Emphasize the significance of personal autonomy in decision-making while prioritizing maternal and fetal well-being, fostering a balance between personal choices and health considerations.

7. Continual Engagement and Education:
- Promote continual engagement in learning and staying updated on the latest research findings and healthcare guidelines to facilitate ongoing informed decision-making.

Empowering pregnant individuals through knowledge equips them to make informed choices regarding cannabis use during pregnancy. By emphasizing access to reliable information, open communication with healthcare providers, exploring alternatives, understanding individual contexts, accessing supportive resources, and promoting continual education, individuals can make decisions aligned with their health priorities while navigating the complexities of cannabis use during gestation.

- <u>Final Thoughts: Emphasizing the importance of seeking professional guidance and support</u>

1. Healthcare Expertise:
- Professional healthcare guidance is invaluable in providing evidence-based information, tailored advice, and comprehensive support concerning cannabis use during pregnancy.

2. Risk Assessment and Management:

- Healthcare professionals play a crucial role in assessing individual risks, offering guidance on potential consequences, and implementing strategies to manage or mitigate potential risks to maternal and fetal health.

3. Personalized Support and Care:
   - Seeking professional support ensures access to personalized care that considers individual circumstances, providing a supportive environment for informed decision-making.

4. Monitoring and Follow-ups:
   - Regular monitoring and follow-ups with healthcare providers allow for ongoing assessment, adjustment of strategies, and addressing concerns or challenges that may arise during pregnancy.

5. Access to Resources and Interventions:
   - Healthcare guidance facilitates access to resources, interventions, or specialized care services designed to support pregnant individuals in reducing or abstaining from cannabis use during gestation.

6. Continual Education and Updates:
   - Healthcare professionals offer continual education, updates on the latest research, and guidance aligned with evolving healthcare practices, ensuring individuals have the most current information for decision-making.

7. Promoting Maternal and Fetal Well-being:
   - Seeking professional guidance prioritizes the well-being of both the pregnant individual and their unborn child, ensuring informed choices that align with optimal health outcomes.

The significance of seeking professional guidance and support from healthcare providers cannot be overstated when navigating decisions regarding cannabis use during pregnancy. Their expertise, personalized care, access to resources, continual monitoring, and commitment to promoting maternal and fetal well-being are essential pillars in making informed and health-conscious decisions throughout the gestational journey.